PROSTATE PROBLEMS:

Safe, Simple, Effective Relief

William Campbell Douglass, MD

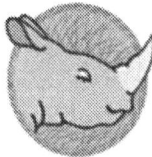

Rhino Publishing, S.A.

PROSTATE PROBLEMS:

Safe, Simple, Effective Relief

ISBN 9962-636-32-9

Cover illustration by
Alex Manyoma (alex@3dcity.com)

Please, visit Rhino's website for other publications from
Dr. William Campbell Douglass
www.rhinopublish.com

Dr. Douglass' "Real Health" alternative medical
newsletter is available at www.realhealthnews.com

RHINO PUBLISHING, S.A.
World Trade Center
Panama, Republic of Panama

Voicemail/Fax
International: + 416-352-5126
North America: 888-317-6767

Contents

Other Books by
William Campbell Douglass, MD

- *Add 10 Years To Your Life*
- *Aids And Biological Warfare*
- *Bad Medicine*
- *Color Me Healthy*
- *Dangerous Legal Drugs: The Poisons In Your Medicine Chest*
- *Dr. Douglass Complete Guide To Better Vision*
- *Eat Your Cholesterol! -- Meat, Milk, And Butter -- And Live Longer*
- *Grandma Bell's A To Z Guide To Healing*
- *Hormone Replacement Therapies: Astonishing Results For Men And Women.*
- *Hydrogen Peroxide - Medical Miracle*
- *Into The Light - Tomorrow's Medicine Today*
- *Lethal Injections - Why Immunizations Don't Work*
- *Painful Dilemma -- Patients In Pain -- People In Prison*
- *Prostate Problems: Safe, Simple Effective Relief*
- *St. Petersburg Nights*
- *Stop Aging Or Slow The Process: Exercise With Oxygen Therapy*
- *The Eagle's Feather*
- *The Joy Of Mature Sex And How To Be A Better Lover...*
- *The Smoker's Paradox: The Health Benefits Of Tobacco*

Section 1

Problems of the Prostate

Justice Harry Blackman of the Supreme Court was out dancing the polka with his wife a few weeks ago. He is 85 years old and was diagnosed with cancer of the prostate in 1987. I tell you this not to prove that only the good die young (although the evidence of that is compelling), but to allay your fears somewhat about cancer of the prostate.

There is no area in medicine where you'll find a greater state of controversy than the treatment of prostate disease, both cancer of the gland and the condition called benign prostatic hypertrophy (BPH).

The controversy is centered around facts indicating that a poor outcome, with many unpleasant and debilitating side effects, is apparently far more common following prostate surgery than the medical authorities have led us to believe.

Presenting his findings at a meeting of the American Society of Clinical Oncology, Dr. James

Talcott of the Dana-Farber Cancer Center, found in a study of 282 patients that a year after their prostate surgery, 41 percent of them had to wear diapers because of chronic leaking from their bladder. Eightyeight percent were finished sexually because of total impotence.

Because surgery has produced such poor results (and also because of the slow-growing nature of this type of cancer), there is now serious debate as to whether the disease should even be diagnosed, much less treated. Although thousands of people who suffer from prostate cancer die yearly, most of them die of other causes before their cancer ever becomes a serious problem. By stirring things up with unnecessary surgery, it's even possible (I think it's *likely*) that many productive years of life may be wasted.

As Dr. Talcott remarked: "Patients need to know what they are in for. We need to prepare them for the bad things that may befall them." Unfortunately, very few physicians are following his advice. That's why this report is so crucial.

Despite the high prevalence of BPH, it may surprise you to learn that, until recently, there has not been any serious attempt to determine the natural history of the disease, i.e., what happens if there is no treatment given at all? This is one reason for the controversy over when, if at all, we should "treat" it.

New federal guidelines are even urging

urologists to curtail the use of two widely employed diagnostic tests, X-ray and ultrasound, and rely instead on a simple seven-item questionnaire. According to the guidelines, the X-ray and ultrasound tests add nothing to the decision as to what type of treatment should be used. A survey in 1989 revealed that two-thirds of urologists routinely use these tests, which add tens of millions of dollars to the overall cost of medicine every year. The questionnaire is designed to ascertain *the quality of life* of the patient. This helps the doctor respond to the *needs of the patient* rather than to cold and impartial laboratory findings, which may be scientifically marvelous, but tell him nothing about how the patient is responding to the problem.

You know the old saying about death and taxes — the two things in this life we can be sure of. But for American men age 50 and over, I must, unfortunately, add another certainty: prostate problems.

It is not my intention to alarm you and, unlike the National Cancer Institute (NCI) and the American Cancer Society (ACS), I'm not predicting that one-third or two-thirds of American men will eventually be diagnosed with prostate cancer. While this may be true, such statistics are misleading as well as self-serving. (If so many men will get prostate cancer, don't we need to allocate more money to the National Cancer Institute?)

My caveat about prostate problems is meant only to make you aware of the potential difficulties all men face. For most men, the problems will be minor—an increased need to urinate or an increased urge to urinate. For others, the problem may involve a decline in sexual performance. I'm not making light of this problem, but it certainly isn't cancer.

Unfortunately, for some prostate cancer is a fatal disease. But in most cases the cancer is not as serious as it sounds. The majority of men with prostate cancer are older—in their late 70s or early 80s. Fortunately, the cancer is usually slow-growing, so that most men die of natural causes well before the prostate cancer becomes a medical problem.

An Enlarged Prostate

If you are experiencing some of the symptoms of an enlarged prostate (BPH), you are most likely suffering from the inconvenience and the worry that cancer is imminent or that sex is a thing of the past. Don't panic; neither may be true.

Let's take a look at how the prostate functions and what you can do to improve the condition of the prostate and relieve the symptoms of BPH—*without dangerous drugs or surgery.*

First, you must understand that *BPH is not an indication of prostate cancer.* Also, BPH *symptoms* are not a precursor to prostate cancer, nor does BPH increase your chances of getting prostate cancer. BPH is worry enough without worrying about something it isn't — and it isn't cancer. If you have any symptoms of BPH, they are indicators of nothing other than an enlarged prostate. To make this important point perfectly clear, let me state it another way: If you have benign prostatic hypertrophy (BPH) your odds of having cancer of the prostate are no higher than anyone else (except, of course, your wife —whose odds are zero).

How the Prostate Works

As part of the male reproductive system, the prostate sits just in front of the rectum and directly under the bladder. The gland encircles the urethra— the tube through which urine passes down the penis and on to the fireplug. If the prostate enlarges, it can squeeze that tube, causing slow and frequent urination.

What exactly does the prostate do? From what we can gather, its main purpose is to add fluid to sperm during sexual intercourse. The fluid helps to power sperm and protect it from the acidic environment of the vaginal canal. It's surprising that with sex being such an important aspect of life so little is known about the physiology of the male sex glands—the epididymis, the testicles, the seminal vesicles, and the prostate gland.

The prostate is in a continual state of growth throughout a man's life. Naturally, the growth begins during puberty, but it undergoes a second stage of growth at age 25.

Even conservative doctors admit that BPH is rarely a problem before age 40, and is mostly a problem much later in a man's life. One statistic— which I hesitate to use—is that 90% of men over age 70 will have some symptoms of BPH. Again, most often those symptoms are not serious in nature and can be remedied without drug therapy—or the need to see a doctor.

In spite of these facts and an admission that BPH isn't much of a problem until later in life, urologists still perform more than 350,000 surgeries for BPH each year. I believe that many of these surgeries are not needed and lead to a lot of unnecessary suffering in an age group that suffers enough without the help of the medical profession.

If the prostate does enlarge, a series of dominolike effects will usually take place: the gland will push against the urethra, which may irritate the bladder wall. The bladder may begin contracting with just a small amount of urine present. Urination will then increase and the bladder will eventually enlarge, become thin-walled, and weaken. A weak bladder cannot fully empty itself—urine remains and the cycle starts again. The stagnant urine in the bladder can also lead to a chronic infection, which further aggravates the problem and puts a strain on the immune system.

Just what causes BPH is not really known. Nor is there any valid information about risk groups or risk factors. A while back, there were a few studies indicating that American men were more likely to suffer from BPH than citizens of other countries. But other reviews have been inconclusive. A few surveys demonstrated that married men had a greater risk, but again, that has never been confirmed.

There are certain risk factors associated with BPH:

* Being over 50 years old

* The taking of some antihypertensive drugs

* Low socioeconomic status

* Low body mass

* Alkaline urine

* Tuberculosis

* A history of bladder or kidney infections

* Professional bachelorhood (Although, and this is an important point, there is *no relation* between sexual activity and BPH. Put another way: "too much" sex or "too little" sex plays *no role* in this disease.)

And certain protective factors:

* Coffee has a weak protective effect

* So does daily alcohol consumption, with beer having the strongest protective effect

* *All studies have found smoking to be negatively associated with prostate surgery.* Strange as it seems, smokers are less likely to end up having prostate operations. As nicotine elevates testosterone levels, this consistent finding is hard to rationalize and I do not recommend that you take up smoking as a BPH preventive. Besides, if you smoke you'll probably die from some other cancer before you're old enough to worry about prostate problems.

One way to avoid all prostate problems is to have your testicles removed before you reach maturity. That's a bit extreme, but it points to that fact the testosterone and/or estrogen—which are produced by the testes—may play a role in BPH and other more serious prostate problems. Yes, men do produce a small amount of estrogen. And as men age the amount of testosterone decreases, leading some to suggest that the increased estrogen levels are the cause of prostate problems. But this theory is just that—a theory which is interesting, but unproven.

Another theory involves a hormone called dihydrotestosterone (DHT), a substance which may control prostate growth. Yet another theory suggests that BPH is controlled by instructions given to the cells at a very early age. Later in life these cells "come to life," so to speak, and give the signal for further prostate growth.

Dihydrotestosterone is a variant of testosterone and it seems to be the hormone that induces hypertrophy (swelling) of the prostate gland. Administration of DHT to beagle dogs induces prostate hypertrophy and, if you inhibit a certain enzyme that is responsible for the conversion of testosterone to DHT, studies in humans have shown that *prostatic hypertrophy* can be reversed. The levels of testosterone do not change with the enzyme inhibition, so the reduction of swelling of the prostate can be assumed to be from decreasing the circulating level of DHT.

You should know the name of the enzyme that we are interested in inhibiting, because we will come back to it when discussing treatment of BPH. It's called five-alpha-reductase (5AR). This is very important, because if you have too much 5AR, you will have too much DHT. And thus you are almost certain to have an enlarged prostate in time.

You now know more about the etiology of benign prostatic hypertrophy than virtually every proctologist and psychiatrist in the universe. DHT and 5AR are not the whole story, and there is much more to be learned. Makes you wonder, then, how medical science can be so certain about treating prostate problems when they don't even understand the cause. It's been my experience that if you don't know the cause of a disease, your treatment often goes awry.

The Symptoms of BPH

As most older men know through personal experience, the symptoms of either BPH or a prostate infection involve an increased need to urinate, particularly at night, leaking, dribbling, and a slowstarting or interrupted stream. If you are experiencing any of these symptoms, there's a good chance that BPH is the cause.

What's worrisome about BPH is that the severity of the symptoms is not indicative of the degree of BPH. Some men have a very swollen prostate, yet have few symptoms. Others can have a mild case of BPH, with little swelling, but still have severe symptoms.

One important warning: If you are experiencing some symptoms, no matter how minor, avoid over-the-counter cold and flu medicines. These drugs can cause acute urinary retention—that is, the inability to urinate at all.

Other things to avoid are alcohol, cold temperatures, and becoming a couch potato. If there's a partial obstruction, these can increase your problem. So, stop drinking and start exercising—a short walk can do wonders for an enlarged prostate.

Other symptoms of BPH can be much more serious. BPH can eventually weaken the bladder, cause urinary tract infections, bladder stones, and kidney problems due to back pressure from the obstruction. Eventually, there will be incontinence in most cases. Once the bladder is damaged, medical science is hard pressed to offer any help.

If You Go to the Doctor

I don't suggest running to the doctor at the first sign of an enlarged prostate, but if you are experiencing symptoms of BPH and are concerned, it may be wise to visit a urologist. Before you make such a visit, I strongly suggest that you try some natural remedies before you give the urologist your hard-earned money (see the **Action to Take** section starting on page 30). Of course, if your problem appears acute—inability to urinate, pain, swelling at the lower abdomen above the pubic bone—you should see a urologist immediately.

Normally, the doctor will perform one or more tests to determine if indeed your prostate is enlarged or infected. The traditional test—and the bane of jokes worldwide—is the digital rectal exam. The doctor inserts a gloved finger into the rectum and feels the prostate. This procedure is as ancient as medicine, but it is not very helpful. When correlated with the findings at surgery, this procedure has been found to be very inaccurate as to the estimation of the size of the prostate.

Some urologists will then suggest an ultrasound exam of the prostate. I don't believe this is necessary in the large majority of cases, but like most things in contemporary medicine, doctors no longer trust their instincts so they depend on "sophisticated" instruments. During the ultrasound exam, a probe is inserted in the rectum and using sound waves— much like radar — an image of the prostate is displayed on a computer monitor. This method is well-correlated with the findings of gland size at surgery, *but there is no correlation with the severity of the bladder outflow obstruction,* so the test is generally not indicated.

It's important to summarize the relevance of prostate size and enlargement to the action taken to treat and, hopefully, cure your problem: There is no relevance to prostate size and subsequent treatment, and all tests done to that end are a waste of time and money.

Another procedure is the urine flow study. The patient is asked to urinate into a device which measures the speed of urine flow. If there's an obstruction, the urine flow will be decreased. *But a slow urine flow does not necessarily mean that you need surgery.* A little more patience maybe, but not necessarily surgery. An excellent monograph on this disease from the Johns Hopkins University School of Hygiene and Public Health states unequivocally: "Urine flow rate alone cannot be used to ... predict favorable response to prostatectomy."

Two other procedures which can be an aid in diagnosis, but are usually not necessary, are the intravenous pyelogram (IVP) and cystoscopy. In the former, dye is injected and an X-ray photo of the urinary tract is taken. The IVP may help in the diagnosis, but it is done primarily to rule out any damage to the kidneys. But injecting dye into your veins can be dangerous. Your doctor may not tell you about the dangers, but let me tell you that serious complications can result from such a procedure. Problems can occur if too much dye is used or if your body has a bad reaction to the dye. The IVP is a time-tested and often useful test when used in hospitals or clinics where they are prepared to treat allergic reactions which, fortunately, are not common —but, they are not rare, either.

Cyctoscopy, where a small tube is inserted through the penis, via the urethra, allows the doctor to see the condition of the bladder. This test can often yield very useful information about the condition of your bladder. Although a local anesthetic is used to numb the inside of the penis, this procedure still hurts.

If BPH is the diagnosis, your doctor will suggest

various treatments. Some more enlightened doctors may suggest a simple but very effective prostate massage. This used to be the preferred method of treatment many years ago, and it often helps. But something as simple as a massage (a process very much like the digital rectal exam, where the physician inserts a gloved finger into the rectum, then massages the prostate) is no longer in vogue. Today we need machines to diagnose and esoteric drug therapies to treat.

Do not let your physician give you nafarelin acetate! This powerful drug is meant to block testosterone production by altering the pituitary gland and, in theory, reduce the size of the swollen prostate. But the research is shaky. Once you stop taking the drug, the prostate returns to its original size, so I assume you're meant to take this drug indefinitely. And do you really want to take a drug that alters your pituitary function?

The side effects of lowering testosterone and/or taking this drug long-term have not been determined. In other words, stay away from this "latest and greatest" solution to BPH.

Prostate Infections

Many times, problems with the prostate are caused by an infection, and not by BPH or cancer. There are several microorganisms that can cause a prostate infection. They enter through the urethra, at the end of the penis, and can cause some painful problems. These germs include coliform bacteria, Staphylococcus, chlamydia, gonorrhea, vaginal yeast, and even tuberculosis—in rare cases.

Almost 90 percent of prostate infections are the coliform variety, with staph germs coming in second.

Coliform bacteria enter through the urethra and can cause infections in the urethra itself, spreading to the prostate and bladder. The causes are many, but can include poor personal hygiene—not washing your hands after exposure to feces, for example. Uncircumcised men must be particularly vigilant when it comes to cleaning the penis.

Sex also plays a role. Prostate infections are greater in men who have multiple sexual partners. And unprotected anal intercourse is an almost sure-fire way to catch a coliform infection.

If you're diagnosed with an infection, your physician will probably prescribe an antibacterial agent, such as a sulfa drug. The most commonly prescribed are Bactrim and Septra. If you are taking these, I recommend that in addition you increase your intake of garlic. As an antibacterial agent garlic is second to none. The equivalent of one clove of garlic per day—of either Kwai or Kyolic tablets— should be the *minimum* intake.

Staphylococcus infections can be tougher to treat,

particularly if the infection was contracted in the hospital. There are drug-resistant strains of staph that can be difficult to treat, and some can be downright deadly.

Gonorrheal prostatitis is sexually transmitted. You may not know that gonorrhea is still very common. Unfortunately, most of us have forgotten about it since AIDS came on the scene. Gonorrhea can be treated with antibiotics, but there are strains that have grown antibiotic resistant.

Don't ignore gonorrhea symptoms (a yellow discharge from the penis, and a sensitive penis tip). Often these symptoms go away, but the gonorrhea remains and can attack other parts of the body. One of my most satisfying diagnoses was in a young black male who came into the emergency room complaining of acute swelling and pain in his joints. This was unusual and so I tested him for gonorrhea. He was positive, including fluid from one of his swollen joints. If he had not been promptly diagnosed and treated, he could have been crippled for life.

I also mentioned TB: Yes, it's back and with a vengeance. TB of the prostate, although still rare, will certainly make a comeback as TB rates continue to rise. TB reaches the prostate through the bloodstream or lymph ducts, just like the gonorrhea in the joints mentioned above. You don't have to engage in sex with an infected individual to contract TB of the prostate. TB is airborne—a cough or sneeze in your direction from an infected person is all you need. Treatment for this type of prostate infection is prolonged, lasting up to one year.

Finally, prostate infections caused by vaginal yeast are common. The symptoms include a mild rash near the groin or an itch inside the penis. The treatment includes antifungal drugs and antifungal topical creams.

One of the most common sources of prostate and bladder infection is from the catheter used following surgery. The organisms travel up the drainage tube from the container hanging on the side of the bed. If doctors would only follow my advice on this problem, I am convinced that most of these infections could be avoided. All they need to do is instruct the nurse to put about 50 mls of three-percent hydrogen peroxide in the collecting bag or bottle and change it frequently, preferably hourly. The doctor just has to write the order on the patient's chart. Is that asking too much? (Most don't do it.)

In *all* of these infections, phototherapy (photoluminescence) should be tried before antibiotics. (See my book, *Into the Light*.)

BPH, Surgery, and Sex

Let's repeat it one more time: *The most recent studies indicate that the best treatment for BPH is often no treatment at all*. This startling conclusion was published in the *Journal of the American Medical Association* after studies showed that most symptoms of BPH *will go away by themselves* if left alone—no surgery, no drugs, no nothing. Just wait, and the chances are very good that your symptoms will disappear just as quickly as they came. Of course, the AMA suggests yearly checkups for men over 50, but these are not necessary if you are symptom-free.

Why then do physicians push for a surgical solution? One reason is *money*. Each year, in spite of the strong evidence that doing nothing is best, more than 350,000 surgeries are performed to treat BPH. The cost of these treatments is in excess of $5 billion. That's a lot of money and as long as worried men are willing to undergo the surgery, physicians will continue to reap the profits.

One source recommends treatment if BPH "causes a major inconvenience." What's a major inconvenience? I'll tell you: months of painful recovery and potential impotence caused by unnecessary surgery, with a depleted bank account. *That's* a major inconvenience.

I understand the psychological and physical problems related to BPH and I know that no matter what I say, some of you will ultimately decide to have surgery in hopes of relieving prostate problems. *But surgery should be the last resort.* Do not let your doctor push you to a surgical solution. In most cases it is not necessary and can create its own set of serious, long-term problems.

There is a "dirty little secret" concerning prostate surgery that you should know about. It's a subterfuge that plays nicely into the hands of any urologist who is willing to deal in the crime of omission—omission in the sense that he's not telling you everything.

With an enlarged prostate, the patient immediately thinks of cancer. As we have explained, there is no relation between BPH and cancer of the prostate. But even if there were, *prostate cancer typically involves a part of the prostate not removed by transurethal resection of the prostate, or TUR.* So don't be panicked into the operation by the "excisional biopsy" ploy— two for the price of one: we are curing your BPH and, at the same time, taking care of any cancer that may be present.

Prostate surgery is uncertain. There's the risk of infection from the surgery (iatrogenic infection, that is, infections you catch in the hospital, are dangerous, and often deadly), the extended period of healing, the cost of surgery, and the possibility of complications, to name just a few.

And of primary concern is the risk of reduced sexual function. Some doctors will tell you that BPH surgery doesn't affect sexual ability. That's just not true. A *conservative* estimate is that sexual function is adversely affected in at least 30 percent of cases. I argue that the figure is nearer 60 percent.

Sure, they'll tell you that after a few months your ability to have sex will return, but that's a ruse. I've seen the few months turn into a year, then two, then ... forget it. I've always believed in the old adage, use it or lose it. For a man in his late fifties or early sixties, a year without sex could lead to a lifetime without sex.

I keep reading that "in time, most men will be able to enjoy sex again." That's what the urologists will tell you. They just never mention that the "time" may be extended well beyond the normal recovery time for the surgery. It's made to sound like a sure thing—but it's not. Are you willing to risk your sex life by undergoing surgery for BPH? That's the first question I'd answer before considering the knife.

The first and most serious potential problem is the inability to maintain an erection. The prostate is in a delicate area of the male anatomy—a place where muscle tissue and blood vessels feeding the penis are abundant. If during surgery muscle is damaged, there's a very good chance of impotence. Can the damage be reversed? Maybe yes, maybe no. And how long it will take to strengthen the damaged muscles is anyone's guess.

For younger men, prostate surgery can make you sterile. I won't go into the physiology, but the bottom line is that semen is no longer ejaculated through the penis. There is often a reverse ejaculation into the bladder. No semen, no ability to impregnate.

Finally, in some cases, men who have had prostate surgery lose their ability to reach sexual climax. Again, doctors will tell you this ability will return in time. Whose time? When?

My suggestion for anything short of prostate cancer, and even then only in the most extreme cases: *Do not have prostate surgery.* The risks are too great; and problems created by the surgery can be permanent.

A Continuing Treatment Dilemma

If you're having to consider prostate surgery, here's a depressing report on the so-called benefits of prostate surgery. A poor outcome, with many unpleasant and debilitating side effects, is apparently far more common following prostate surgery than the surgeons have led us to believe.

Presenting his findings at a meeting of the American Society of Clinical Oncology, Dr. James Talcott, of the Dana-Farber Cancer Center, found in a study of 282 patients that a year after their prostate surgery, 41 percent of the patients had to wear diapers because of a chronic leak from the bladder. Eighty-eight percent were finished sexually because of total impotence.

The surgery has produced such poor results, and because of the slow-growing nature of this type of cancer, it is now seriously debated as to whether the disease should even be diagnosed, much less treated. Although thousands die of prostate cancer yearly, most of them die of other causes before the cancer ever becomes a problem. By stirring things up with surgery, many good, productive years of life may be wasted.

As Dr. Talcott remarked: "Patients need to know what they are in for. We need to prepare them for the bad things that may befall them."

Types of Surgery

For your information, I've outlined the types of surgery most commonly used for BPH. *This is for your information only.* If your doctor suggests "transurethral surgery," for instance, at least you'll know what the procedure entails and that you probably don't want it.

The most common type of surgery for BPH is called transurethral resection of the prostate, or TUR. A 12-inch resectoscope is inserted into the penis through the urethra. The "scope" includes a mechanism for cutting prostate tissue and sealing the blood vessels.

TUR surgery takes nearly two hours. The supposed benefit (if there is any benefit at all) is that no incision is needed. Also, the time of recovery is much less than with other types of prostate surgery and there are fewer complications. This is what we were taught in medical school and this is what the patients are told, but it has proven not to be true.

Many recent studies have found *consistently higher rates of postoperative mortality and higher re-operation rates* with transurethral prostatectomies, TUR, as compared with open prostatectomies (discussed below). These studies were reported in some of the finest medical journals in the world: the *British Medical Journal*, the journal *Prostate*, and the *Journal of Urology*. Yet, most urologists cling to the TUR procedure and ignore the evidence that they are putting their patients at unnecessary risk of death or a failed operation that will *again* subject them to the same risk.

Another type of prostate surgery is called transurethral *incision*. The process involves cutting at the point where the bladder joins the urethra and widening the urethra. Many physicians argue that this surgery has fewer side effects than TUR. That's interesting, since most claim TUR has no side effects to begin with. From what I've seen, the transurethral incision is unproven and potentially dangerous.

The newest and most expensive technique uses a laser to literally vaporize the prostate tissue that is causing the obstruction. But again, this technique is new and is far from proven. And don't let anyone fool you—*laser surgery is still surgery. There is pain and the potential for serious side effects.*

Finally, there's the old stand-by—open surgery.

Here, the chances of damaging muscle and blood vessels feeding the penis are great. Once damaged, you can just about forget your sex life. And an open incision under anesthetic presents the potential for serious problems, including staph infections and a reaction to the anesthesia, either of which could be fatal. But, contrary to what we were told in medical school, the old open method is still preferred *although 95 percent of BPH is still treated by transurethral resection.*

After any of the above surgeries, there is a period of recovery that requires a hospital stay. When discharged, you may have a catheter in the penis for awhile. These are very uncomfortable, subject to infection, and often cause very painful spasms of the bladder.

On top of that, there's a regimen of antibiotics you will have to take to avoid the dreaded infection from killer hospital super bugs. And, for a while, your urine will run red, as blood, including clots, is passed in the urine.

Does any of this sound like a minor inconvenience? That's what most docs will tell you, but you will find out that there's nothing minor about bladder pain and catheters.

There are a few other possible side effects of surgery. Once the catheter is removed, you may still feel the urgency to urinate. (Wasn't that one of the symptoms surgery was supposed to relieve?)

Urination could be painful for two months or longer.

In some cases, you won't be able to control your bladder at all. That means it's time for Depends, and that time could continue for several months, until the bladder finally heals, or indefinitely.

Open surgery also can produce many of the same problems I've already mentioned related to sex: failure to maintain an erection, impotence, sterility, inability to experience an orgasm, and retrograde ejaculation.

One further point: surgery often does not work. The prostate can become enlarged again, requiring even more surgery. And occasionally, the scar tissue left behind by surgery needs to be surgically removed — sometimes surgery begets surgery.

The Other Side of the Coin

Having now frightened you into a state of urinary incontinence, I must tell you that BPH, in some men, can have serious consequences if not treated. These include diverticula (pits) in the bladder which can lead to infection, bladder stones, hydronephrosis (a ballooning of the kidneys resulting in renal failure and death), and acute retention of urine.

This latter complication, acute urinary retention, is *unpredictable in onset* and men who develop it *tend not to be those with the most complaints*. In fact this distressing situation, the inability to pass urine and a consequent swollen and painful bladder, may be the first sign of BPH. In other words, all of us old-timers are sitting on a time bomb. If this happens, believe me, the urologist will be your best friend.

Nonsurgical Treatments

The ineffectiveness of BPH surgery, and the public's reluctance to undergo the unproven ordeal, has led to development of so-called advanced nonsurgical techniques.

I have to admire the tenacity of some physicians. They tell you that surgery is needed and that the side effects are minimal. Then a few years later they tell you surgery isn't needed because there's a new technique that has fewer side effects. Wait a minute. Didn't you just say that surgery had few side effects? So now we have fewer than few side effects?

The three most touted nonsurgical techniques for BPH are balloon urethroplasty, transurethral hyperthermia, and various drug treatments.

Balloon urethroplasty, much like the famous (and questionable) heart treatment called angioplasty, involves a thin tube containing an expandable balloon. The tube is inserted into the opening of the penis and the balloon is then inflated. The theory is that the balloon will expand the urethra and make it easier for urine to pass.

Certainly this will relieve the symptoms of BPH, but for how long? The angioplasty technique for clogged arteries (inserting a balloon into the arteries to push open arterial plaque) has been disappointing and only temporarily effective. The technique itself is dangerous, but studies have shown that the opened arteries soon close again: sometimes in less than three months.

I suggest that this same failure awaits balloon urethroplasty. The urethra will be forced open, but in a matter of months it will again narrow, perhaps even more than before the procedure. You'll experience the same symptoms and you'll have to go through the procedure one more time. At an additional cost, I might add. My advice: pass on urethroplasty.

Transurethral hyperthermia is the new darling of the urology world. Here, heat is applied directly to the prostate via a catheter inserted into the urethra. The heat is supposed to shrink the prostate. The side effects of this procedure are very similar to those of surgery: irritation of the urethra, bleeding, and those very painful bladder spasms. No studies have proven its effectiveness, so why undergo the procedure if it's unproven? And, like any other assault on part of your body, there are potential side effects. This method *may* be the best yet devised, but we'll have to wait and see.

Finally, drug companies are scrambling to be the first to "discover" a treatment for BPH. But to date, not even the AMA is recommending any drug therapy for BPH. (Even the medical bureaucracy gets it right once in a while. But I predict that pressure from their favorite advertisers will help them see the light eventually.)

Drug companies don't give up, particularly when there's so much money to be gained from men over age 50. Think of it: if a drug gets AMA and FDA approval, it will most likely be prescribed to almost every male at one time or another during his lifetime. That's a large, multi-billion dollar market just waiting to happen.

Some companies are concentrating their efforts on "alpha adrenergic blockers." Currently used (overused, I should say) to treat high blood pressure, some believe these drugs can reduce enlarged prostates. The generic drug names are phenoxybenzamine, prazosin, and terazosin. One such drug, marketed as Hytrin, has been submitted by Abbott Labs to the FDA for approval. And many urologists are already prescribing the drug for BPH. I'll give them an "A" for independence, but an "F" for judgement.

There's no proof that Hytrin does anything other than treat the symptoms of BPH. It does not reduce an enlarged prostate, and the long-term effects of Hytrin are not known. Here's the irony: blood pressure medication is notorious for causing impotence in males. Doctors will prescribe a drug that supposedly helps fight BPH, but at the same time causes one of the more serious symptoms of BPH— impotence. I don't know about you, but if the cure for BPH is impotence, I'll suffer the symptoms of an enlarged prostate. At your age, you can do without that kind of help.

And, since Hytrin is used to treat high blood pressure, what happens if your blood pressure is fine? You take Hytrin to treat BPH and your blood pressure drops, perhaps to a dangerously low level. My advice is to run, don't walk, away from any doctor prescribing Hytrin or other alpha adrenergic blockers to treat BPH.

Earlier I spoke about drugs that control testosterone and their use to treat BPH. There is a history of using these drugs, especially estrogen, the female hormone, to treat BPH. But the side effects of such drugs include the same effects you'll find from castration! Men taking estrogen suffer from impotence, loss of sexual drive, loss of energy, and, in extreme cases, the development of female physical characteristics, including rather impressive breasts. Okay, men, who wants to be the first to try these drugs?

The newest testosterone-lowering drug to be touted by the pharmaceutical industry is Proscar. The theory is that there is "good" testosterone and "bad" testosterone. There's testosterone and dihydro-testosterone (DHT). The latter is critical during puberty. Scientists tell us that DHT is bad for older men and, from your science lesson above, you will no doubt concur. So doctors are now prescribing Proscar, which prevents (good) testosterone from converting into (bad) DHT.

This sounds great and the theory of good and bad can feed off the anti-cholesterol craze with its good (HDL) and bad (LDL) forms of cholesterol. The makers of Proscar, Merck & Co., admit that the drug takes at least six months to work and can cause impotence. But, in fact, studies reported in the *New England Journal of Medicine* indicate that Proscar *doesn't work at all.* There is also a possibility that the drug is carcinogenic. Wouldn't that be something? A "cure," approved by the FDA, that gives you cancer.

But here's the really sleazy part of this story: Saw palmetto berries, in the form of an extract called LSE seronoa, are just as effective as Proscar in inhibiting the conversion of testosterone to DHT, maybe more so. The herb is nontoxic and costs a third as much as Merck's drug. But the Food and Drug Administration rejected an application to have the extract approved as an over-the-counter treatment for BPH. Although the saw palmetto extract has been used for BPH since 1905, and is listed in all the pharmacopeias, the *Physician's Desk Reference* (until 1948, when it was quietly removed), and all the pharmacy texts, the FDA declared the herb to be an "unapproved new drug"!

Action to Take

(1) If you have a prostate problem, but there is no blockage to the flow of urine, or if the blockage is not so bad that you can't live with it, forego surgery. You can always have surgery, but you can't undo what has been done. It's not like getting a haircut.

(2) Get some saw palmetto berries and make a tea out of them (weak at first to test your sensitivity, then gradually increase the strength) or make an "infusion" (prolonged soaking in water) and keep it refrigerated. Drink the tea or the infusion, one cupful, three times a day.

There is scientific evidence for this treatment. Saw palmetto berries inhibit the enzyme 5-alpha-reductase, and a low activity of this enzyme is associated with a reduced risk of prostate cancer. This berry is also effective in the treatment of benign prostatic hypertrophy, which is not always so "benign" in its effects.

(3) Although it may sound a little strange if you are having difficulty urinating, force yourself to drink a lot of fluids and eat a lot of watermelon. I can't guarantee that this will cure your problem, but it might and the least it will do is discourage bladder infection by increasing urine flow. Drink six to eight glasses of water daily.

(4) Parsley has been considered a "prostate herbal" for

years. Make a tea from the leaves (the stronger the better). Add lemon for taste.

(5) Some common-sense things to do:

* Limit fluid intake in the evening.

* Avoid long intervals between urination; *plan ahead,* especially for travel.

    With each urination, empty the bladder as fully as possible.

* Be alert to the possibility of infection. If you have any burning, frequency, or cloudy urine, see a urologist right away.

See the end of the cancer section for further suggestions on the natural therapy of prostate disease and information about a support group.

Section 2

Prostate Cancer

You have probably heard the medical warnings about prostate cancer: it's the third most prevalent type of cancer in America and the second most common among men (skin cancer is first). Some statistics indicate that one man in ten will get cancer of the prostate and the number of cases is growing. One estimate is that 200,000 new cases of prostate cancer are diagnosed each year.

Yet, with all this disease being presented to doctors, the specialists are sharply divided on what treatment is best. As you might expect, the surgeons are not too enthusiastic about the trend toward a wait-and-see approach to cancer of the prostate. The surgeons may not like it, but this approach is gaining ground because *no studies have been completed, that experts agree on, that show surgery or radiation provides any survival advantage over waiting.* Large-scale studies are underway, but the answer, if any, is at least ten years in the future.

Those researchers defending a more conservative approach point out that the survival rates from radical surgical treatment and radiation for *localized* prostate cancer are no better than those obtained by the conservatives who gave their patients *no initial treatment at all.*

One obvious point that many overlook is that the number of cases has increased because men are living longer. Yes, if you live to be 85 or 90 or beyond, chances are you'll have some form of prostate cancer. Chances are you'll have heart disease, too. And I'll bet you'll need glasses and will probably walk with a limp. But these conditions are part of living longer and are not related to a relative increase in the incidence of the disease. Would you treat a 50year-old for a heart condition that *may* develop into something serious when he is an octogenarian? That's the theory used by many urologists to justify the treatment of *potential* metastatic prostate cancer.

The most important point is that in *most cases* prostate cancer is slow-growing and in no way shortens life or limits sexual activity. That's why medical journals, like the *Journal of the American Medical*

Association, are now telling us that the best treatment *is no treatment at all.*

A small cancer in the prostate may, and usually will, stay within the confines of the gland for many years. Surgery in these slow-moving cancers is not only unnecessary, but is actually contraindicated and dangerous. Surgery can be *fatal* due to blood clots, infection, or metastatic spread from the surgery itself.

Don't let your doctor frighten you into quick surgery. If you have cancer of the prostate, a few weeks of contemplation is not going to endanger your life. Get a second, or even a third opinion. (Note: Get the second opinion in another town. Doctors have to live together and don't want to offend their colleagues by saying a surgical procedure is unnecessary.)

I do have to warn you that there are some forms of prostate cancer that move quickly and can be deadly. We'll list the symptoms of serious prostate cancer a little later so you'll know what to look for and how to proceed.

There are a few theories about the causes of prostate cancer. These theories range from repressed sexual behavior (one study indicates that sexual repression causes a buildup of male hormones in the prostate that eventually cause cancer), to a high fat diet, to vasectomies (some studies indicate a greater risk of prostate cancer in men who have had vasectomies). None of these theories are proven and I don't have one of my own other than processed foods, smoking, and the inevitable increase in cancer as we age.

Age *is* the greatest risk factor for prostate cancer. Under age 50, prostate cancer is rare, and more than 80 percent of all diagnosed cases are in men over age 65.

The Four Stages of Prostate Cancer

Prostate cancer is divided into four stages—"A" through "D." If you go to your physician and he starts talking about Stage A or Stage B, you should be armed with some information about what he means.

Stage A cancer means the malignant tumor is confined within the prostate itself. This type of cancer is almost impossible to diagnose, even with the much-heralded prostate specific antigen test (PSA). Urologists hope that a new diagnostic technique will be developed so that Stage A cancers can be detected. I hope not. Finding prostate cancer at such an early stage is a curse, not a blessing. In many instances, the cancer, if left alone, will never progress. *But* if you start treating these early cancers—start poking and sticking them—you just about *guarantee* that the cancers will grow. If you have Stage A cancer of the prostate you probably don't know it, and your doctor doesn't need to know either. *There are no symptoms indicating Stage A.*

Stage B prostate cancer indicates that a detectable

tumor has been found within the prostate but is still confined to it. Most of these cancers are discovered by the traditional digital rectal exam. There are substages within Stage B: B-1 means the tumor is in one lobe of the prostate only and is small in size (less than 3/4 in.); B-2 means the tumor is in two lobes, or is greater than 3/4 in. *The symptoms for Stage B include all of those related to prostatic hypertrophy (BPH):* frequent urination, an increased urgency to urinate, and a reduced or broken stream. But there's a chance you may not have any symptoms at all.

Stage C cancer indicates that the tumor is no longer confined to the prostate. Usually the malignancy has moved from the prostate to the testicles. During Stage C, symptoms may increase. They include those symptoms mentioned for Stage B, plus pain in the area of the prostate.

Stage D prostate cancer is the end of the road for most patients. The cancer has metastasized, that is, the cancer has spread throughout the body. Symptoms may include serious problems urinating, significant weight loss, and pain in the bones around the pelvis, the lower back, and the upper thighs.

Blood Tests

To determine if your problems are related to cancer of the prostate, your doctor may perform a blood test.

The most popular and the newest is the PSA, or *prostate specific antigen* test. In theory the test checks your blood for levels of a protein which is found in the prostate gland only. Again, in theory, when the level of this protein is above normal, prostate cancer is likely.

I'm not against the test, *per se,* but it does present some problems. First, PSA has shown a great deal of inaccuracy. False positives *and* false negatives have been reported. So no matter what the results of the PSA test, you can't be certain.

But what bothers me the most is the fact that a positive test will get your doctor moving in the direction of treatment—probably surgery. And for most cases of prostate cancer, surgery or drug therapies are not needed. The cancer may be so small as to be insignificant. But by the time your doctor gets finished with his poking and prodding, you can bet the cancer will have grown.

Let me repeat what I've said many times in this report: The AMA itself is now saying that in *most cases,* the best thing to do with prostate problems— including BPH and cancer—is *nothing.* Symptoms of BPH often disappear on their own; cancer of the prostate is usually slow moving and may not grow at all. For most men, prostate cancer is not a killer, nor does it significantly shorten your life.

If cancer is detected, your doctor may then order a prostate acid phosphate test (PAP). This test determines if the cancer has spread throughout the body.

How Prostate Cancer Is Treated

Again, let me repeat that in most cases the best way to treat prostate problems, including most cancers, is to do nothing. This goes double for men over age 65. The chances that the cancer will kill you are minimal. Prostate cancer is slow growing, in most cases.

But if you have been diagnosed as Stage C or worse (and you've had a second opinion), then action is necessary. *But that action does not have to include surgery.* There are alternatives — such as photoluminescence therapy and treatment with hydrogen peroxide. Cutting and burning are the *very last* alternatives in most cases. At this stage, hormones may help relieve the misery of this terminal condition and so may radiation treatment. However, the doctor and the patient are now fighting a losing battle and the objective should be to make the patient as pain-free as possible. With modern pain management, there is no excuse for anybody in a modern society to die in pain.

If a tumor has been discovered, *under no circumstances should you permit your doctor to perform a needle biopsy on the tumor. Such a biopsy can only help to spread the cancer throughout your system.* A needle, no matter how small, is basically a knife, and when the needle passes into the gland, it is cutting tissue which, if cancer is present, can spread the tumor. A cancer which is localized in the prostate is a problem, but it can be controlled. Once the cancer branches out, your chances of survival drop to below 20 percent.

Traditional medicine will treat prostate cancer either with surgery or with radiation treatment. I'm against both—but not always. There are times when removal of the prostate can eliminate the cancer completely. Yes, the procedure may cause impotence, but which would you prefer: a healthy sex life limited to a few years, or a long, celibate life with good books, good company, and good wine? As I grow toward maturity, the choice is becoming more clear.

If you are under age 60, removing a cancerous prostate can add decades to your life—again, in some cases. But the cost of a radical prostatectomy is almost always impotence and incontinence.

Other types of surgery, including the use of lasers, have been tried, but found to be ineffective because they fail to remove all of the cancer. But work continues on surgical methods that will remove the cancer without causing impotence and/or incontinence.

Radiation is the second method of treatment. Quite simply, the prostate is hit with radiation meant to destroy the cancer. One problem: the radiation doesn't know which cells are cancerous and which are not. So it bombards the entire region, killing cancer cells and healthy ones alike. Cells surrounding the prostate are also destroyed. Physicians will tell you that this unintended damage has now been minimized, but don't believe it. And there are other side effects associated with the treatment, ranging from nausea to diarrhea to rectal bleeding.

Another "creative" way to deliver the radiation is to place a radioactive "seed" into the prostate. These seeds contain radioactive materials that, in theory, destroy the cancer from within the prostate. But the seeds continue to emit radiation even after the cancer (and probably the entire prostate area) has been destroyed. As Nancy Reagan used to say: "Just Say No" to radiation therapy.

If I had my choice, and there were no alternatives, I would opt for surgery over radiation, *but only after I was certain the cancer was growing rapidly and that other alternative treatments had been exhausted.*

Taking Care of Your Prostate

Obviously, the best way to avoid surgery is to prevent the problem in the first place. But if you're already having problems, there are two specific changes you can make to improve the condition of your prostate and alleviate symptoms of BPH:

Reduce the use of drugs and use specific vitamins, minerals, and herbs.

Before we discuss drugs, a few common-sense steps to take:

(1) Lose weight. Obesity creates problems of all kinds, particularly prostate problems.

(2) Cut down on your alcohol consumption. Too much alcohol adversely affects a man's sexual performance and alcohol can irritate the prostate. The prostate can contain concentrations of alcohol more than ten times greater than in the bloodstream. Use all things in moderation, including alcohol, especially if you have a prostate problem. *Some* alcohol is good for the prostate, a lot is *bad.*

(3) Start a light exercise program. A sedentary lifestyle isn't good for your body. So start walking. It will give you energy, exercise the prostate, help you lose weight, and can improve your sexual energy and performance.

Now let's discuss drugs and their effects on prostate and sexuality.

As we age, doctors think it's fine to prescribe drug after drug after drug—drugs for high blood pressure, drugs for insomnia, drugs for anxiety, and on and on. Most of these drugs adversely affect your prostate, your sexual drive, and your ability to maintain an erection.

Take a look at the prescription and over-the-counter drugs you are taking. Eliminate as many of these drugs as possible. And I suggest you take a look at my book, *Dangerous (Legal) Drugs.* I wrote this monograph particularly for men and women over age 50. It outlines which drugs are dangerous and lists those that can adversely affect sexuality and your prostate.

Even those over-the-counter drugs which seem benign can irritate the prostate. Foremost among these are antihistamines. In many men, particularly those over age 50, antihistamines play a role in impotence and incontinence. And they adversely affect the prostate and the bladder. What's so insidious about antihistamines is that they are so readily available, and most of us think of them as totally safe. They are not!

Blood pressure medications present more problems, such as impotency and incontinence, plus reduced sexual urge and overall energy. They can also irritate the prostate and increase the symptoms of BPH.

As a simple rule of thumb, most prescription drugs and some over-the-counter drugs have the potential to affect sexuality and the overall condition of your prostate, not to mention the rest of your system. If you suddenly develop symptoms of BPH, there's a good chance a medication is involved— especially if you've just started taking a new medication.

Natural Supplements
and the Health of Your Prostate

If you haven't yet heard, the new hero of the herbal medicine crowd, of which I am a member, is the saw palmetto. This berry has shown an amazing ability to eliminate the symptoms of BPH and reduce the size of an enlarged prostate. In fact, the *British Journal of Pharmacology* reports that the saw palmetto berry *works as well or better than the drug, Proscar,* for reducing an enlarged prostate.

Unfortunately, you won't read much about saw palmetto, because the FDA has ruled it illegal to advertise the herb as a solution to any prostate problem. But take it from me, in many cases saw palmetto is all you need. For an enlarged prostate, I suggest two to three capsules of saw palmetto two to three times a day. This regimen works, but it can take up to six months before you notice the improvement. I think you will agree that six months of taking saw palmetto beats surgery laden with side effects. Once the symptoms of BPH are gone, take one or two capsules once a day to keep your prostate healthy.

Add zinc to your diet. Numerous studies have clearly shown that a zinc deficiency will adversely affect the condition of your prostate. In fact, the prostate contains a higher concentration of zinc than any other organ in the body. If you are on one of those low red-meat, low-calorie diets, the chances are good that you're low in zinc. The best source of the mineral is red meat. Eat your meat and take 25 mg to 50 mg of zinc each day.

Note: if you are taking an iron supplement, absorption of zinc is compromised. So you may want to reduce or eliminate iron supplementation.

Take a magnesium supplement. Along with protecting your heart, magnesium has been shown to protect the urinary system and to prevent the formation of kidney stones. How magnesium works is not known, but it can help your heart. Take 250 mg to 500 mg each day.

Selenium is another element that can help improve sexuality and the condition of your prostate. Selenium helps to regulate the level of male hormones and thus plays a role in maintaining a healthy prostate and a vigorous sex life. I suggest 100 mcg to 200 mcg each day.

An herb that helps to relieve the symptoms of BPH is the juniper berry. This herb is a powerful diuretic and there's some evidence it can help the prostate. Juniper berry is available at most health food stores. Make sure you take only the amount recommended by the manufacturer. Too much juniper can irritate the urinary tract.

Pumpkin seed oil has also shown promise in

improving the prostate. Some experts claim that prostate problems can be worsened by the presence of parasitic worms in the lower intestine. Pumpkin seed oil kills these worms.

Linus Pauling, who was treated for prostate cancer, recommends vitamin C for an enlarged prostate. He could be right. I don't know, but taking 500 mg of C each day can't hurt, and it just might help.

I've read some preliminary reports that show bee pollen works well to improve the condition of the prostate and increase sexual energy. Some claim bee pollen can reduce an enlarged prostate. However, if you are allergic to bee stings *do not* use bee pollen. There have been reports of dangerous allergic reactions in some people using bee pollen.

Finally, some in the natural health field are touting the ability of vitamin F to reduce BPH and eliminate the need for surgery. Vitamin F, linoleic, and linolenic acids, have been used for prostate problems and as a preventive against kidney damage. But the case for vitamin F is not conclusive. If you are suffering from the first signs of an enlarged prostate, trying vitamin F and tracking the progress of your symptoms would be worth the effort.

If you have a prostate problem, either BPH or cancer, I recommend that you contact the Patient Advocates for Advanced Treatment (PAAT). PAAT is the world's largest prostate cancer organization and is dedicated to the detection, diagnosis, evaluation, and treatment of prostate cancer. You can contact this non-profit organization by calling (616) 453-1477 or writing PAAT, 1143 Parmelee NW, Grand Rapids, Michigan 49504-3844. Any contributions would be greatly appreciated.

With the many conflicting reports—and even the urologists being at odds with each other—on how to treat cancer of the prostate and BPH, we may have helped "confuse you with the facts." But this, unfortunately, is the nature of the beast. You need to know all your options, even when they're contradictory. Spoon-feeding you or short-changing you will only lead to bad decisions.

Take your time; don't be rushed into surgery or any other form of treatment.

Index

About Doctor William Campbell Douglass II

Dr. Douglass reveals medical truths, and deceptions, often at risk of being labeled heretical. He is consumed by a passion for living a long healthy life, and wants his readers to share that passion. Their health and well-being comes first. He is anti-dogmatic, and unwavering in his dedication to improve the quality of life of his readers. He has been called "the conscience of modern medicine," a "medical maverick," and has been voted "Doctor of the Year" by the National Health Federation. His medical experiences are far reaching-from battling malaria in Central America - to fighting deadly epidemics at his own health clinic in Africa - to flying with U.S. Navy crews as a flight surgeon - to working for 10 years in emergency medicine here in the States. These learning experiences, not to mention his keen storytelling ability and wit, make Dr. Douglass' newsletters (Daily Dose and Real Health) and books uniquely interesting and fun to read. He shares his no-frills, no-bull approach to health care, often amazing his readers by telling them to ignore many widely-hyped good-health practices (like staying away from red meat, avoiding coffee, and eating like a bird), and start living again by eating REAL food, taking some inexpensive supplements, and doing the pleasurable things that make life livable. Readers get all this, plus they learn how to burn fat, prevent cancer, boost libido, and so much more. And, Dr. Douglass is not afraid to challenge the latest studies that come out, and share the real story with his readers. Dr. William C. Douglass has led a colorful, rebellious, and crusading life. Not many physicians would dare put their professional reputations on the line as many times as this courageous healer has. A vocal opponent of "business-as-usual" medicine, Dr. Douglass has championed patients' rights and physician commitment to wellness throughout his career. This dedicated physician has repeatedly gone far beyond the call of duty in his work to spread the truth about alternative therapies. For a full year, he endured economic and physical hardship to work with physicians at the Pasteur Institute in St. Petersburg, Russia, where advanced research on photoluminescence was being conducted. Dr. Douglass comes from a distinguished family of physicians. He is the fourth generation Douglass to practice medicine, and his son is also a physician. Dr. Douglass graduated from the University of Rochester, the Miami School of Medicine, and the Naval School of Aviation and Space Medicine.

You want to protect those you love from the health dangers the authorities aren't telling you about, and learn the incredible cures that they've scorned and ignored?
Subscribe to the free Daily Dose updates "...the straight scoop about health, medicine, and politics." by sending an e-mail to real_sub@agoramail.net with the word "subscribe" in the subject line.

Dr. William Campbell Douglass'
Real Health:

Had Enough?

Enough turkey burgers and sprouts?

Enough forcing gallons of water down your throat?

Enough exercising until you can barely breathe?

Before you give up everything just because "everyone" says it's healthy...

Learn the facts from Dr. William Campbell Douglass, medicine's most acclaimed myth-buster. In every issue of Dr. Douglass' Real Health newsletter, you'll learn shocking truths about "junk medicine" and how to stay healthy while eating eggs, meat and other foods you love.

With the tips you'll receive from Real Health, you'll see your doctor less, spend a lot less money and be happier and healthier while you're at it. The road to Real Health is actually easier, cheaper and more pleasant than you dared to dream.

Subscribe to Real Health today by calling 1-800-981-7162 or visit the Real Health web site at www.realhealthnews.com.
Use promotional code : DRHBDZZZ

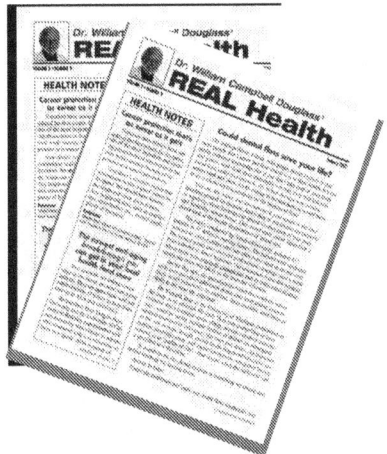

If you knew of a procedure that could save thousands, maybe millions, of people dying from AIDS, cancer, and other dreaded killers....

Would you cover it up?

It's unthinkable that what could be the best solution ever to stopping the world's killer diseases is being ignored, scorned, and rejected. But that is exactly what's happening right now.

The procedure is called "photoluminescence". It's a thoroughly tested, proven therapy that uses the healing power of the light to perform almost miraculous cures.

This remarkable treatment works its incredible cures by stimulating the body's own immune responses. That's why it cures so many ailments--and why it's been especially effective against AIDS! Yet, 50 years ago, it virtually disappeared from the halls of medicine.

Why has this incredible cure been ignored by the medical authorities of this country? You'll find the shocking answer here in the pages of this new edition of Into the Light. Now available with the blood irradiation Instrument Diagram and a complete set of instructions for building your own "Treatment Device". Also includes details on how to use this unique medical instrument.

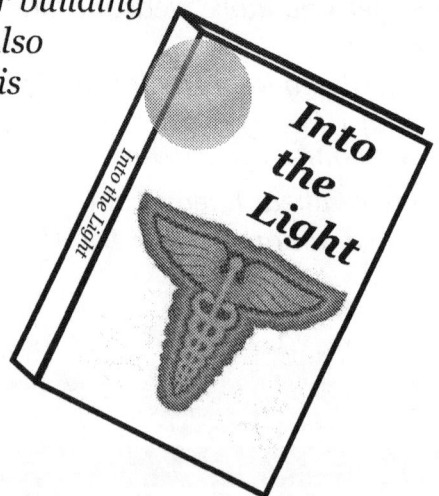

Into the Light

Into the Light

Rhino Publishing S.A.
www.rhinopublish.com

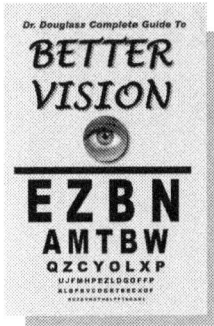

Dr. Douglass' Complete Guide to Better Vision

A report about eyesight and what can be done to improve it naturally. But I've also included information about how the eye works, brief descriptions of various common eye conditions, traditional remedies to eye problems, and a few simple suggestions that may help you maintain your eyesight for years to come. -William Campbell Douglass II, MD

The Hypertension Report. Say Good Bye to High Blood Pressure.

An estimated 50 million Americans have high blood pressure. Often called the "silent killer" because it may not cause symptoms until the patient has suffered serious damage to the arterial system. Diet, exercise, potassium supplements chelation therapy and practically anything but drugs is the way to go and alternatives are discussed in this report.

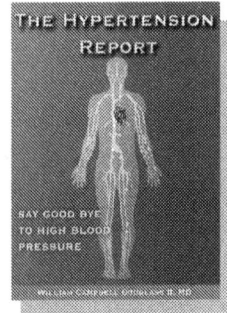

Grandma Bell's A To Z Guide To Healing With Herbs.

This book is all about - coming home. What I once believed to be old wives' tales - stories long destroyed by the new world of science - actually proved to be the best treatment for many of the common ailments you and I suffer through. So I put a few of them together in this book with the sincere hope that Grandma Bell's wisdom will help you recover your common sense, and take responsibility for your own health. -William Campbell Douglass II, MD

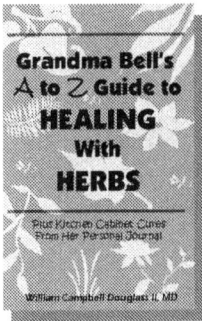

Prostate Problems: Safe, Simple, Effective Relief for Men over 50.

Don't be frightened into surgery or drugs you may not need. First, get the facts about prostate problems... know all your options, so you can make the best decisions. This fully documented report explains the dangers of conventional treatments, and gives you alternatives that could save you more than just money!

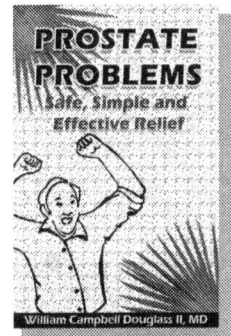

Color me Healthy
The Healing Powers of Colors

"He's crazy!"
"He's got to be a quack!"
"Who gave this guy his medical license?"
"He's a nut case!"

In case you're wondering, those are the reactions you'll probably get if you show your doctor this report. I know the idea of healing many common ailments simply by exposing them to colored light sounds far-fetched, but when you see the evidence, you'll agree that color is truly an amazing medical breakthrough.

When I first heard the stories,
I reacted much the same way.
But the evidence so
convinced me, that I had to
try color therapy in my practice.
My results were truly amazing.

-William Campbell Douglass II, MD

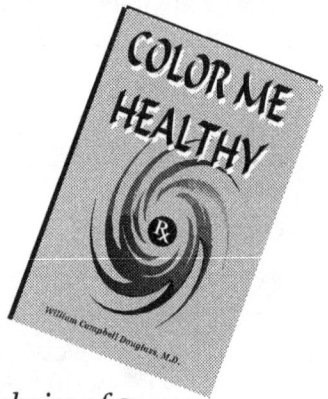

Order your complete set of Roscolene filters (choice of 3 sizes) to be used with the "Color Me Healthy" therapy. The eleven Roscolene filters are # 809, 810, 818, 826, 828, 832, 859, 861, 866, 871, and 877. The filters come with protective separator sheets between each filter. The color names and the Roscolene filter(s) used to produce that particular color, are printed on a card included with the filters and a set of instructions on how to fit them to a lamp.

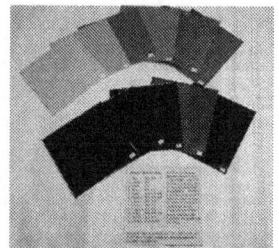

What Is Going on Here?

Peroxides are supposed to be bad for you. Free radicals and all that. But now we hear that hydrogen peroxide is good for us. Hydrogen peroxide will put extra oxygen in your blood. There's no doubt about that. Hydrogen peroxide costs pennies. So if you can get oxygen into the blood cheaply and safely, maybe cancer (which doesn't like oxygen), emphysema, AIDS, and many other terrible diseases can be treated effectively. Intravenous hydrogen peroxide rapidly relieves allergic reactions, influenza symptoms, and acute viral infections.

No one expects to live forever. But we would all like to have a George Burns finish. The prospect of finishing life in a nursing home after abandoning your tricycle in the mobile home park is not appealing. Then comes the loss of control of vital functions the ultimate humiliation. Is life supposed to be from tricycle to tricycle and diaper to diaper? You come into this world crying, but do you have to leave crying? I don't believe you do. And you won't either after you see the evidence. Sounds too good to be true, doesn't it? Read on and decide for yourself.

-William Campbell Douglass II, MD

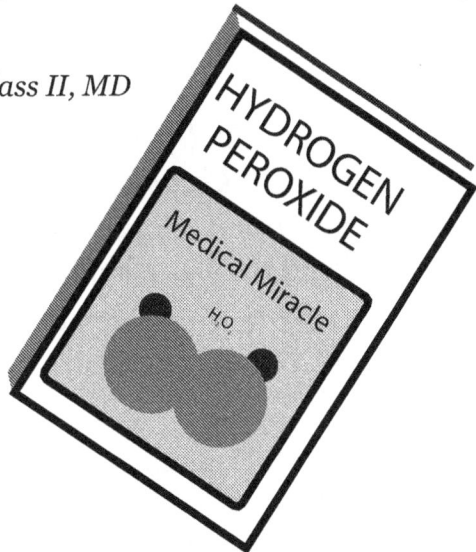

HYDROGEN PEROXIDE

Medical Miracle

H_2O

Don't drink your milk!

If you knew what we know about milk... BLEECHT! All that pasteurization, homogenization and processing is not only cooking all the nutrients right out of your favorite drink. It's also adding toxic levels of vitamin D.

This fascinating book tells the whole story about milk. How it once was nature's perfect food...how "raw," unprocessed milk can heal and boost your immune system ... why you can't buy it legally in this country anymore, and what we could do to change that.

Dr. "Douglass traveled all over the world, tasting all kinds of milk from all kinds of cows, poring over dusty research books in ancient libraries far from home, to write this light-hearted but scientifically sound book.

Rhino Publishing, S.A.
www.rhinopublish.com

The
Milk Book

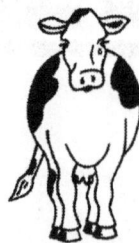

William Campbell Douglass II, MD

Eat Your Cholesterol!

Eat Meat, Drink Milk, Spread The Butter- And Live Longer!
How to Live off the Fat of the Land and Feel Great.

Americans are being saturated with anti-cholesterol propaganda. If you watch very much television, you're probably one of the millions of Americans who now has a terminal case of cholesterol phobia. The propaganda is relentless and is often designed to produce fear and loathing of this worst of all food contaminants. You never hear the food propagandists bragging about their product being fluoride-free or aluminum-free, two of our truly serious food-additive problems. But cholesterol, an essential nutrient, not proven to be harmful in any quantity, is constantly pilloried as a menace to your health. If you don't use corn oil, Fleischmann's margarine, and Egg Beaters, you're going straight to atherosclerosis hell with stroke, heart attack, and premature aging -- and so are your kids. Never feel guilty about what you eat again! Dr. Douglass shows you why red meat, eggs, and dairy products aren't the dietary demons we're told they are. But beware: This scientifically sound report goes against all the "common wisdom" about the foods you should eat. Read with an open mind.

Rhino Publishing, S.A.
www.rhinopublish.com

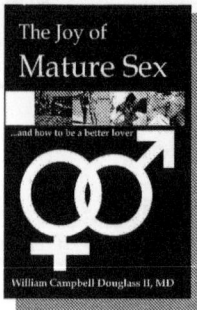

The Joy of Mature Sex and How to Be a Better Lover

Humans are very confused about what makes good sex. But I believe humans have more to offer each other than this total licentiousness common among animals. We're talking about mature sex. The kind of sex that made this country great.

Stop Aging or Slow the Process How Exercise With Oxygen Therapy (EWOT) Can Help

EWOT (pronounced ee-watt) stands for Exercise With Oxygen Therapy. This method of prolonging your life is so simple and you can do it at home at a minimal cost. When your cells don't get enough oxygen, they degenerate and die and so you degenerate and die. It's as simple as that.

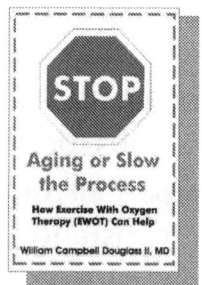

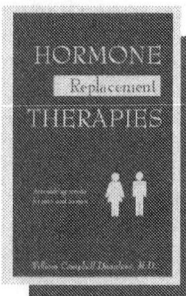

Hormone Replacement Therapies: Astonishing Results For Men And Women

It is accurate to say that when the endocrine glands start to fail, you start to die. We are facing a sea change in longevity and health in the elderly. Now, with the proper supplemental hormones, we can slow the aging process and, in many cases, reverse some of the signs and symptoms of aging.

Add 10 Years to Your Life With some "best of" Dr. Douglass' writings.

To add ten years to your life, you need to have the right attitude about health and an understanding of the health industry and what it's feeding you. Following the established line on many health issues could make you very sick or worse! Achieve dynamic health with this collection of some of the "best of" Dr. Douglass' newsletters.

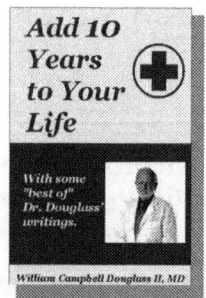

How did AIDS become one of the Greatest Biological Disasters in the History of Mankind?

GET THE FACTS

AIDS and BIOLOGICAL WARFARE covers the history of plagues from the past to today's global confrontation with AIDS, the Prince of Plagues. Completely documented *AIDS and BIOLOGICAL WARFARE* helps you make your own decisions about how to survive in a world ravaged by this horrible plague.

You will learn that AIDS is not a naturally occuring disease process as you have been led to believe, but a man-made biological nightmare that has been unleashed and is now threatening the very existence of human life on the planet.

There is a smokescreen of misinformation clouding the AIDS issue. Now, for the first time, learn the truth about the nature of the crisis our planet faces: its origin -- how AIDS is really transmited and alternatives for treatment. Find out what they are not telling you about AIDS and Biological Warfare, and how to protect yourself and your loved ones. AIDS is a serious problem worldwide, but it is no longer the major threat. You need to know the whole story. To protect yourself, you must know the truth about biological warfare.

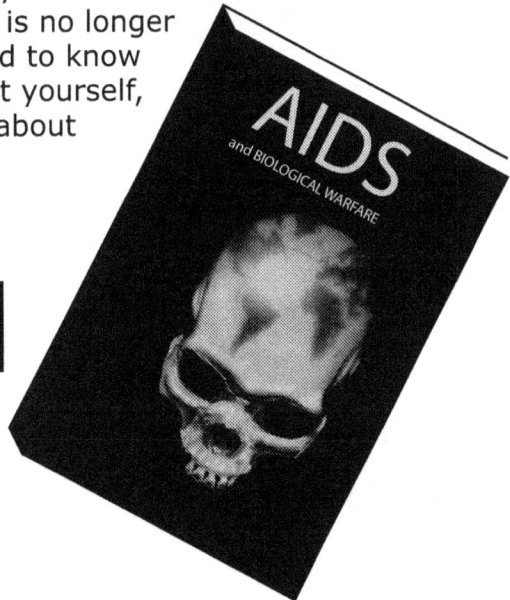

PAINFUL DILEMMA

Are we fighting the wrong war?

We are spending millions on the war against drugs while we
should be fighting the war against pain with those drugs!

As you will read in this book, the war on drugs was lost a long time ago and,
when it comes to the war against pain, pain is winning! An article in USA Today
(11/20/02) reveals that dying patients are not getting relief from pain. It seems
the doctors are torn between fear of the government, certainly justified, and a
clinging to old and out dated ideas about pain, which is NOT justified.

A group called Last Acts, a coalition of health-care groups, has released a very
discouraging study of all 50 states that nearly half of the 1.6 million Americans
living in nursing homes suffer from untreated pain. They said that life was being
extended but it amounted to little more than "extended pain and suffering."

This book offers insight into the history of pain treatment and the current failed
philosophies of contemporary medicine. Plus it describes some of today's most
advanced treatments for alleviating certain kinds of pain. This book is not another
"self-help" book touting home remedies; rather, Painful Dilemma: Patients in
Pain -- People in Prison, takes a hard look at where we've gone wrong and what
we (you) can do to help a loved one who is living with chronic pain.

The second half of this book is a must read if you value your freedom. We now
have the ridiculous and tragic situation of people
in pain living in a government-created hell by
restriction of narcotics and people in prison for
trying to bring pain relief by the selling of
narcotics to the suffering. The end result of the
"war on drugs" has been to create the greatest
and most destructive cartel in history, so great,
in fact, that the drug Mafia now controls most
of the world economy.

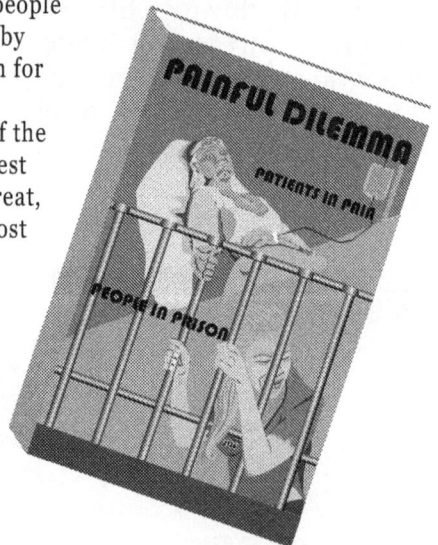

PAINFUL DILEMMA
PATIENTS IN PAIN
PEOPLE IN PRISON

Rhino Publishing S.A.
www.rhinopublish.com

Live the Adventure!

Why would anyone in their right mind put everything they own in storage and move to Russia, of all places?! But when maverick physician Bill Douglass left a profitable medical practice in a peaceful mountaintop town to pursue "pure medical truth".... none of us who know him well was really surprised.

After All, anyone who's braved the outermost reaches of darkest Africa, the mean streets of Johannesburg and New York, and even a trip to Washington to testify before the Senate, wouldn't bat and eye at ducking behind the Iron Curtain for a little medical reconnaissance!

Enjoy this imaginative, funny, dedicated man's tales of wonder and woe as he treks through a year in St. Petersburg, working on a cure for the world's killer diseases. We promise --

YOU WON'T BE BORED!

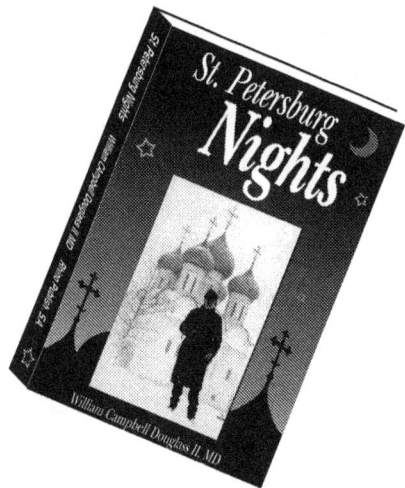

THE SMOKER'S PARADOX
THE HEALTH BENEFITS OF TOBACCO!

The benefits of smoking tobacco have been common knowledge for centuries. From sharpening mental acuity to maintaining optimal weight, the relatively small risks of smoking have always been outweighed by the substantial improvement to mental and physical health. Hysterical attacks on tobacco notwithstanding, smokers always weigh the good against the bad and puff away or quit according to their personal preferences. Now the same anti-tobacco enterprise that has spent billions demonizing the pleasure of smoking is providing additional reasons to smoke. Alzheimer's, Parkinson's, Tourette's Syndrome, even schizophrenia and cocaine addiction are disorders that are alleviated by tobacco. Add in the still inconclusive indication that tobacco helps to prevent colon and prostate cancer and the endorsement for smoking tobacco by the medical establishment is good news for smokers and non-smokers alike. Of course the revelation that tobacco is good for you is ruined by the pharmaceutical industry's plan to substitute the natural and relatively inexpensive tobacco plant with their overpriced and ineffective nicotine substitutions. Still, when all is said and done, the positive revelations regarding tobacco are very good reasons indeed to keep lighting those cigars - but only 4 a day!

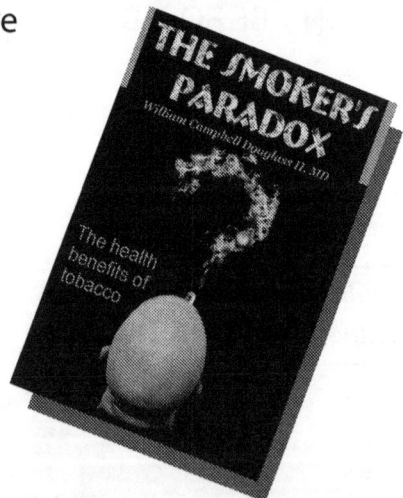

THE SMOKER'S PARADOX

William Campbell Douglass II, MD

The health benefits of tobacco

Rhino Publishing, S.A
www.rhinopublish.com

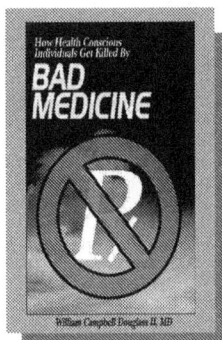

Bad Medicine
How Individuals Get Killed By Bad Medicine.

Do you really need that new prescription or that overnight stay in the hospital? In this report, Dr. Douglass reveals the common medical practices and misconceptions endangering your health. Best of all, he tells you the pointed (but very revealing!) questions your doctor prays you never ask. Interesting medical facts about popular remedies are revealed.

Dangerous Legal Drugs
The Poisons in Your Medicine Chest.

If you knew what we know about the most popular prescription and over-the-counter drugs, you'd be sick. That's why Dr. Douglass wrote this shocking report about the poisons in your medicine chest. He gives you the low-down on different categories of drugs. Everything from painkillers and cold remedies to tranquilizers and powerful cancer drugs.

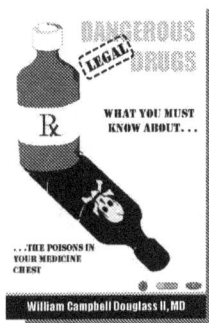

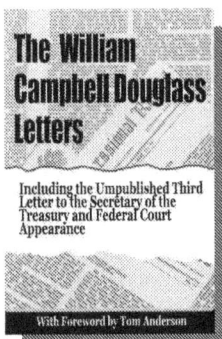

The William Campbell Douglass Letters.
Expose of Government Machinations (Vietnam War).

THE WILLIAM CAMPBELL DOUGLASS LETTERS. Dr. Douglass' Defense in 1968 Tax Case and Expose of Government Machinations during the Vietnam War.

The Eagle's Feather. A Novel of International Political Intrigue.

Although The Eagle's Feather is a work of fiction set in the 1970's, it is built, as with most fiction, on a framework of plausibility and background information. This is a fiction book that could not have been written were it not for various ominous aspects, which pose a clear and present danger to the security of the United States.

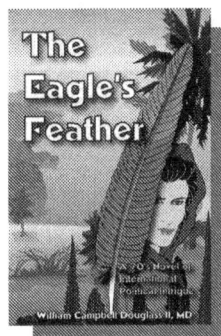

Rhino
Publishing

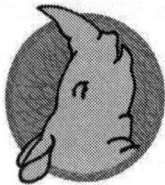

ORDER FORM

PURCHASER INFORMATION

Purchaser's Name (Please Print): _____

Shipping Address (Do not use a P.O. Box): _____

City: _____ State/Prov.: _____ Country: _____

Zip/Postal Code: _____ Telephone No.: _____ Fax No.: _____

E-Mail Address (if interested in receiving free e-Books when available): _____

CREDIT CARD INFO (CIRCLE ONE):

MASTERCARD, VISA, AMERICAN EXPRESS, DISCOVER, JCB, DINER'S CLUB, CARTE BLANCHE.

Charge my Card -> Number #: _____ Exp.: _____

*Security Code: _____ * Required for all MasterCard, Visa and American Express purchases. For your security, we require that you enter your card's verification number. The verification number is also called a CCV number. This code is the 3 digits farthest right in the signature field on the back of your VISA/MC, or the 4 digits to the right on the front of your American Express card. Your credit card statement will show **a different name than Rhino Publishing** as the vendor.

WE DO NOT share your private information, we use 3rd party credit card processing service to process your order only.

ADDITIONAL INFORMATION

If your shipping address is not the same as your credit card billing address, please indicate your card billing address here.

_____   Type of card: _____
Name on the card

Billing Address: _____

City: _____ State/Prov.: _____ Zip/Postal Code: _____

Fax a copy of this order to:
RHINO PUBLISHING, S.A.
1-888-317-6767 or International #: + 416-352-5126

To order by mail, send your payment by first class mail only to the following address. Please include a copy of this order form. Make your check or bank drafts (NO postal money order) payable to RHINO PUBLISHING, S.A. and mail to:

Rhino Publishing, S.A.
Attention: PTY 5048
P.O. Box 025724
Miami, FL.
USA 33102

Digital E-books also available online: www.rhinopublish.com

Rhino
Publishing

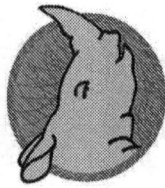

ORDER
FORM

Purchaser's Name (Please Print):

I would like to order the following paperback book of Dr. Douglass (Alternative Medicine Books):

___	X	9962-636-04-3	Add 10 Years to Your Life. With some "best of" Dr. Douglass writings.	$13.99 $_____
___	X	9962-636-07-8	AIDS and Biological Warfare. What They Are Not Telling You!	$17.99 $_____
___	X	9962-636-09-4	Bad Medicine. How Individuals Get Killed By Bad Medicine.	$11.99 $_____
___	X	9962-636-10-8	Color Me Healthy. The Healing Power of Colors.	$11.99 $_____
___	X	9962-636 -XX-X	Color Filters for Color Me Healthy. 11 Basic Roscolene Filters for Lamps.	$21.89 $_____
___	X	9962-636-15-9	Dangerous Legal Drugs. The Poisons in Your Medicine Chest.	$13.99 $_____
___	X	9962-636-18-3	Dr. Douglass' Complete Guide to Better Vision. Improve eyesight naturally.	$11.99 $_____
___	X	9962-636-19-1	Eat Your Cholesterol! How to Live off the Fat of the Land and Feel Great.	$11.99 $_____
___	X	9962-636-12-4	Grandma Bell's A To Z Guide To Healing. Her Kitchen Cabinet Cures.	$14.99 $_____
___	X	9962-636-22-1	Hormone Replacement Therapies. Astonishing Results For Men & Women	$11.99 $_____
___	X	9962-636-25-6	Hydrogen Peroxide: One of the Most Underused Medical Miracle.	$15.99 $_____
___	X	9962-636-27-2	Into the Light. New Edition with Blood Irradiation Instrument Instructions.	$19.99 $_____
___	X	9962-636-54-X	Milk Book. The Classic on the Nutrition of Milk and How to Benefit from it.	$17.99 $_____

	ISBN	Title	Price	
___ X	9962-636-00-0	Painful Dilemma - Patients in Pain - People in Prison.	$17.99	$ _____
___ X	9962-636-32-9	Prostate Problems. Safe, Simple, Effective Relief for Men over 50.	$11.99	$ _____
___ X	9962-636-34-5	St. Petersburg Nights. Enlightening Story of Life and Science in Russia.	$17.99	$ _____
___ X	9962-636-37-X	Stop Aging or Slow the Process. Exercise With Oxygen Therapy Can Help.	$11.99	$ _____
___ X	9962-636-60-4	The Hypertension Report. Say Good Bye to High Blood Pressure.	$11.99	$ _____
___ X	9962-636-48-5	The Joy of Mature Sex and How to Be a Better Lover...	$13.99	$ _____
___ X	9962-636-43-4	The Smoker's Paradox: Health Benefits of Tobacco.	$14.99	$ _____

Political Books:

	ISBN	Title	Price	
___ X	9962-636-40-X	The Eagle's Feather. A 70's Novel of International Political Intrigue.	$15.99	$ _____
___ X	9962-636-46-9	The W. C. D. Letters. Expose of Government Machinations (Vietnam War).	$11.99	$ _____
		SUB-TOTAL:		$ _____

	ADD $5.00 HANDLING FOR YOUR ORDER:		$ 5.00	$ 5.00
___ X	ADD $2.50 SHIPPING FOR EACH ITEM ON ORDER:		$ 2.50	$ _____
	NOTE THAT THE MINIMUM SHIPPING AND HANDLING IS $7.50 FOR 1 BOOK ($5.00 + $2.50)			
	For order shipped outside the US, add $5.00 per item			
___ X	ADD $5.00 S. & H. OR EACH ITEM ON ORDER (INTERNATIONAL ORDERS ONLY)		$ 5.00	$ _____
	Allow up to 21 days for delivery (we will call you about back orders if any)			
		TOTAL:		$ _____

Fax a copy of this order to: 1-888-317-6767 or Int'l + 416-352-5126
or mail to: Rhino Publishing, S.A. Attention: PTY 5048 P.O. Box 025724, Miami, FL., 33102 USA
Digital E-books also available online: www.rhinopublish.com